This Book Belongs To:

____

Color Test Page

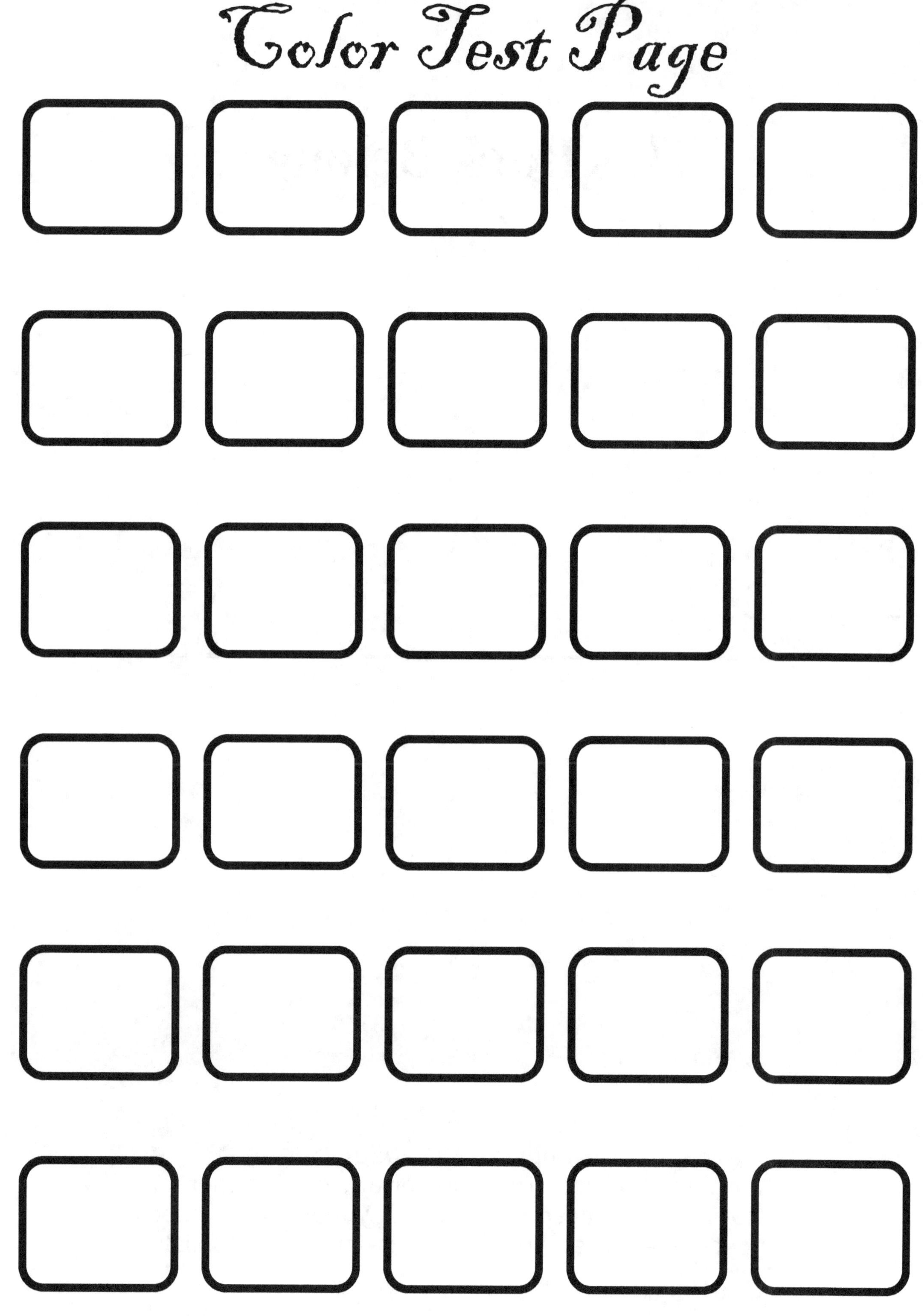

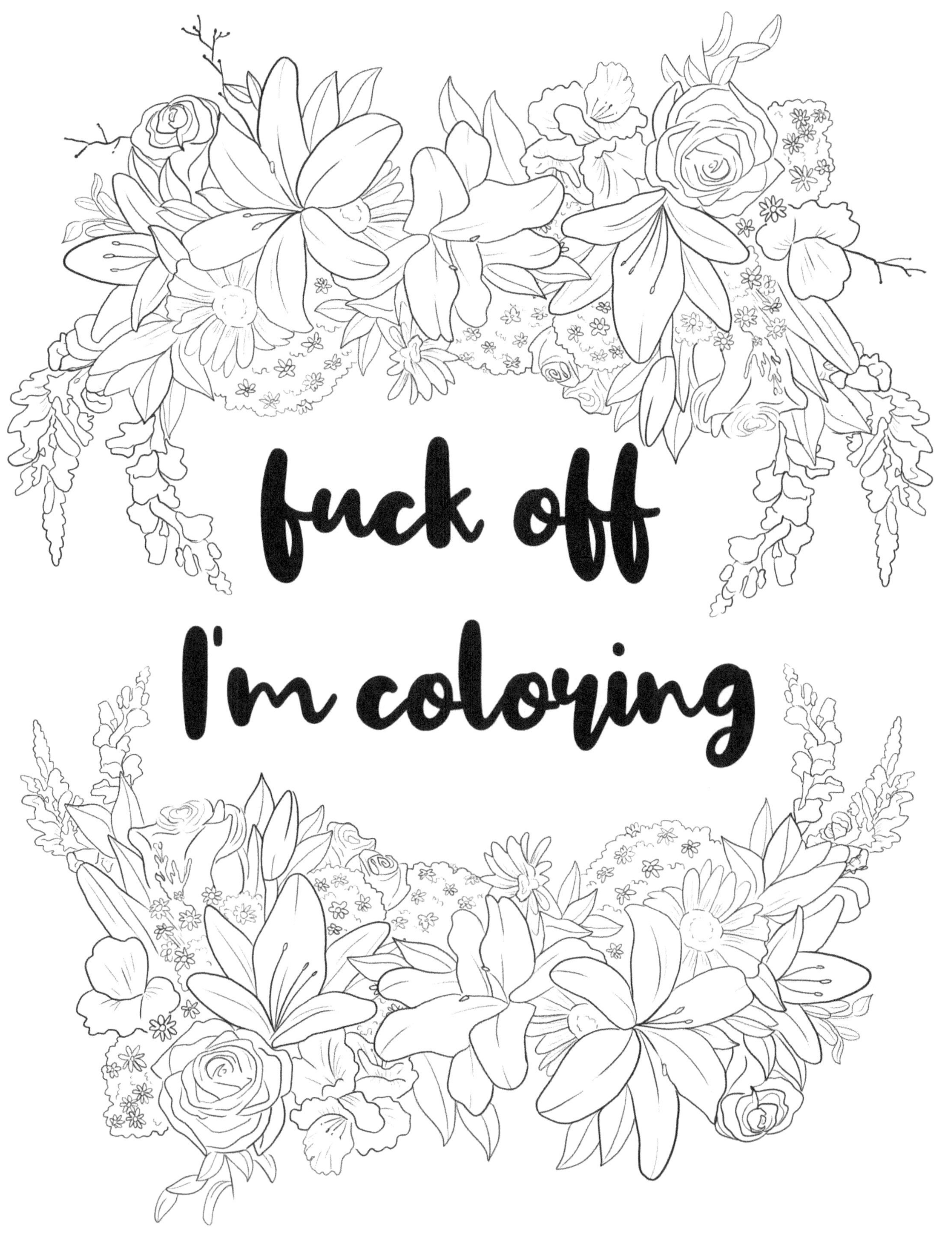
fuck off
I'm coloring

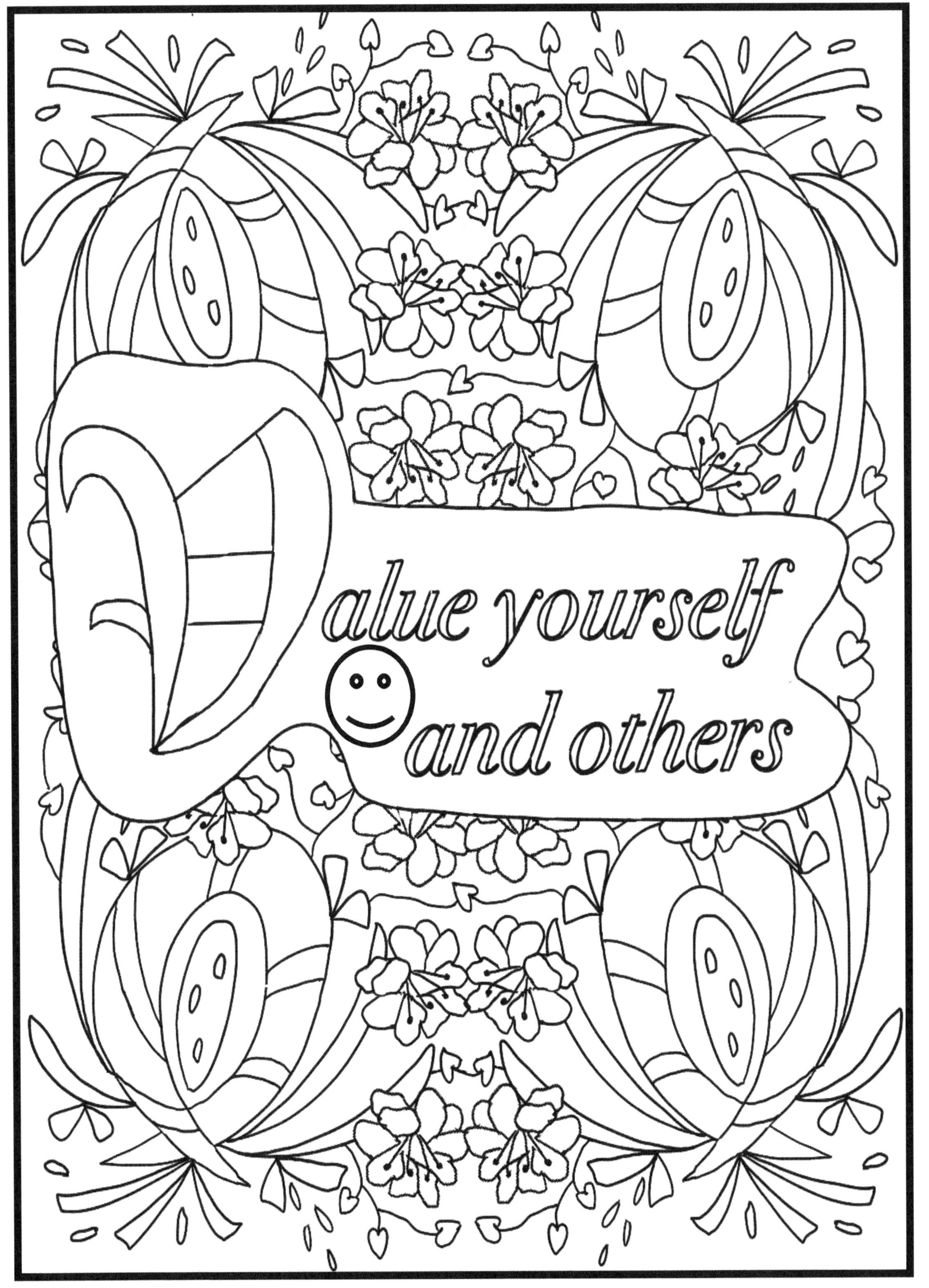

Value yourself
and others

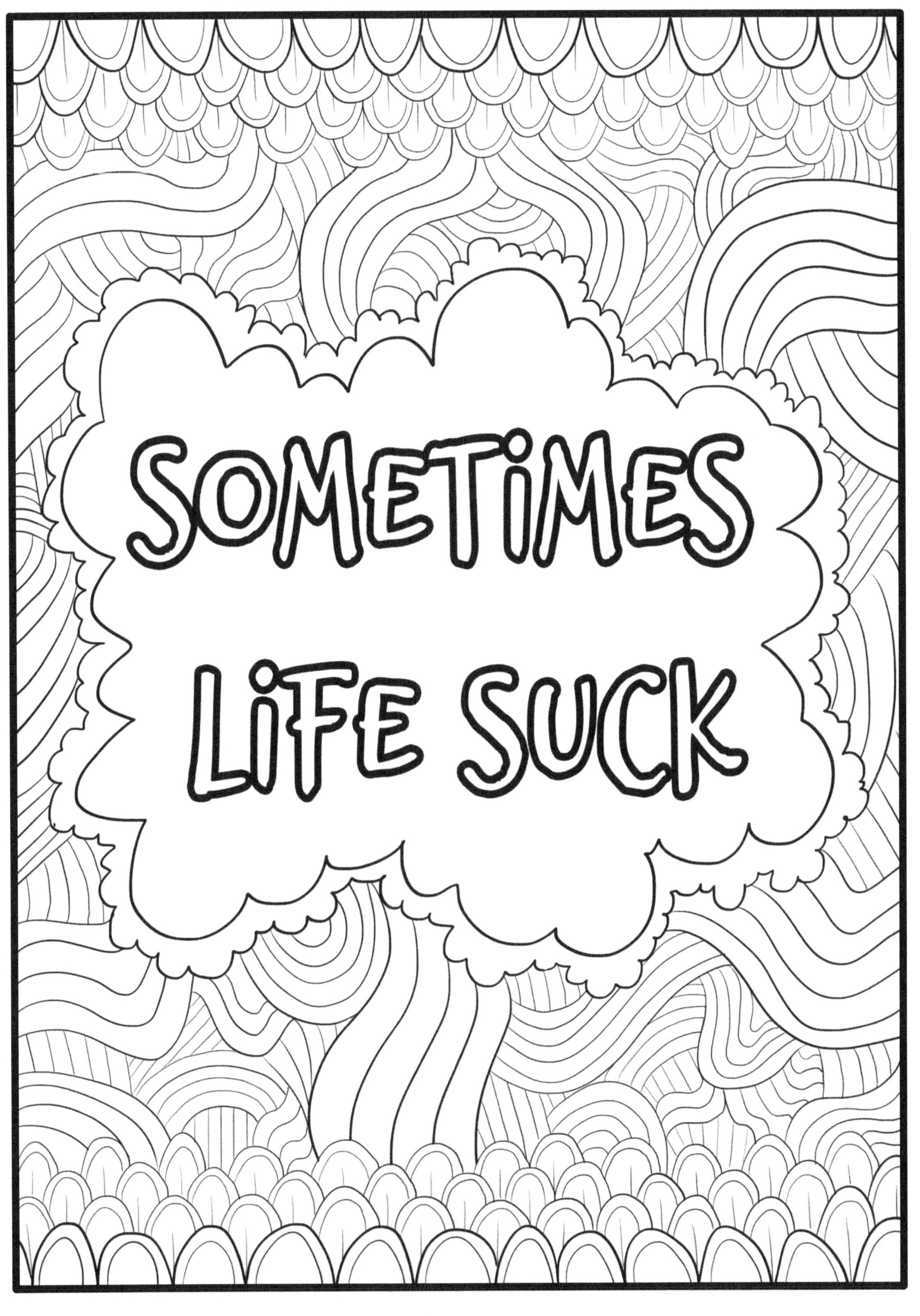

SOMETIMES
LIFE SUCK

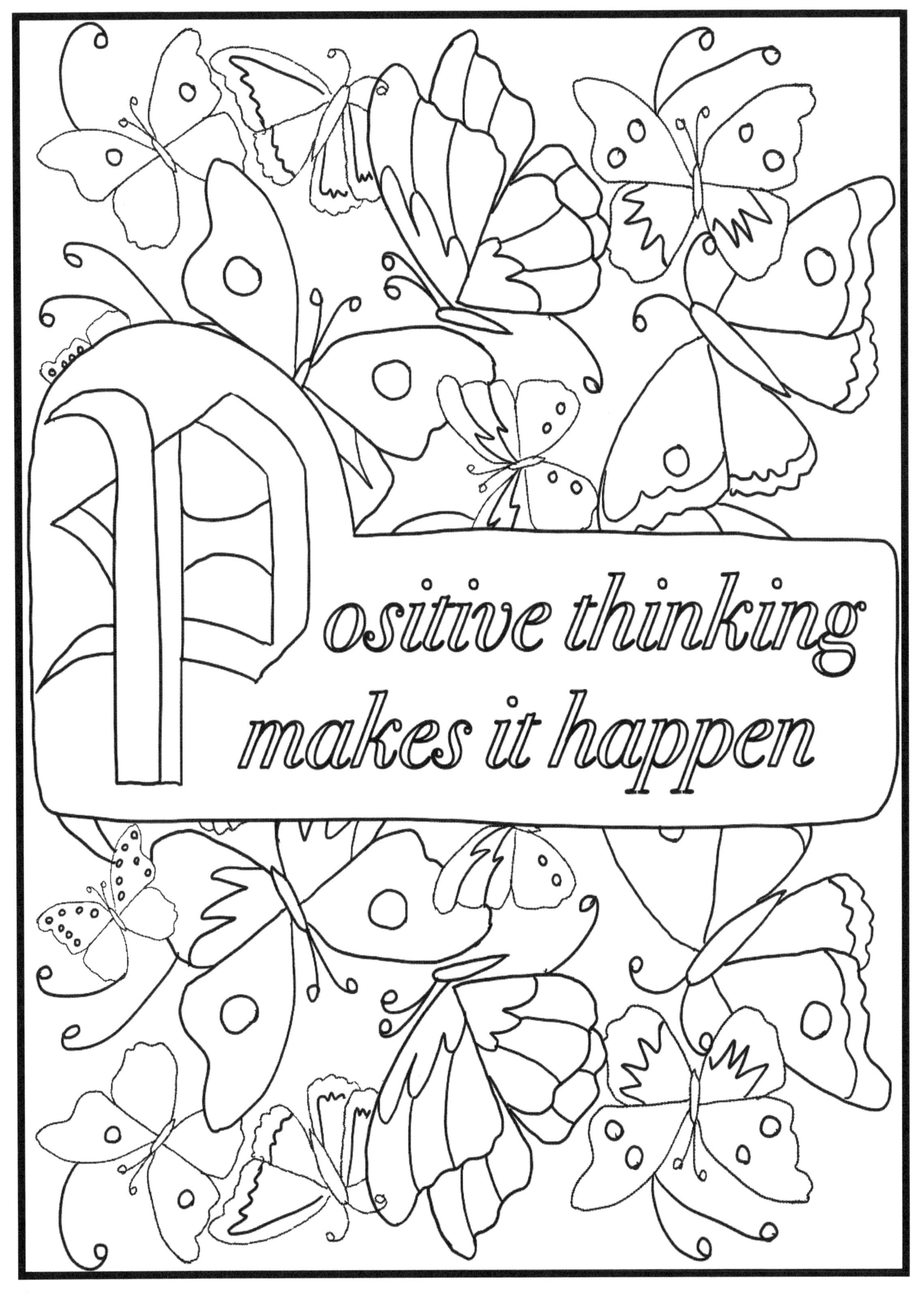

Positive thinking makes it happen

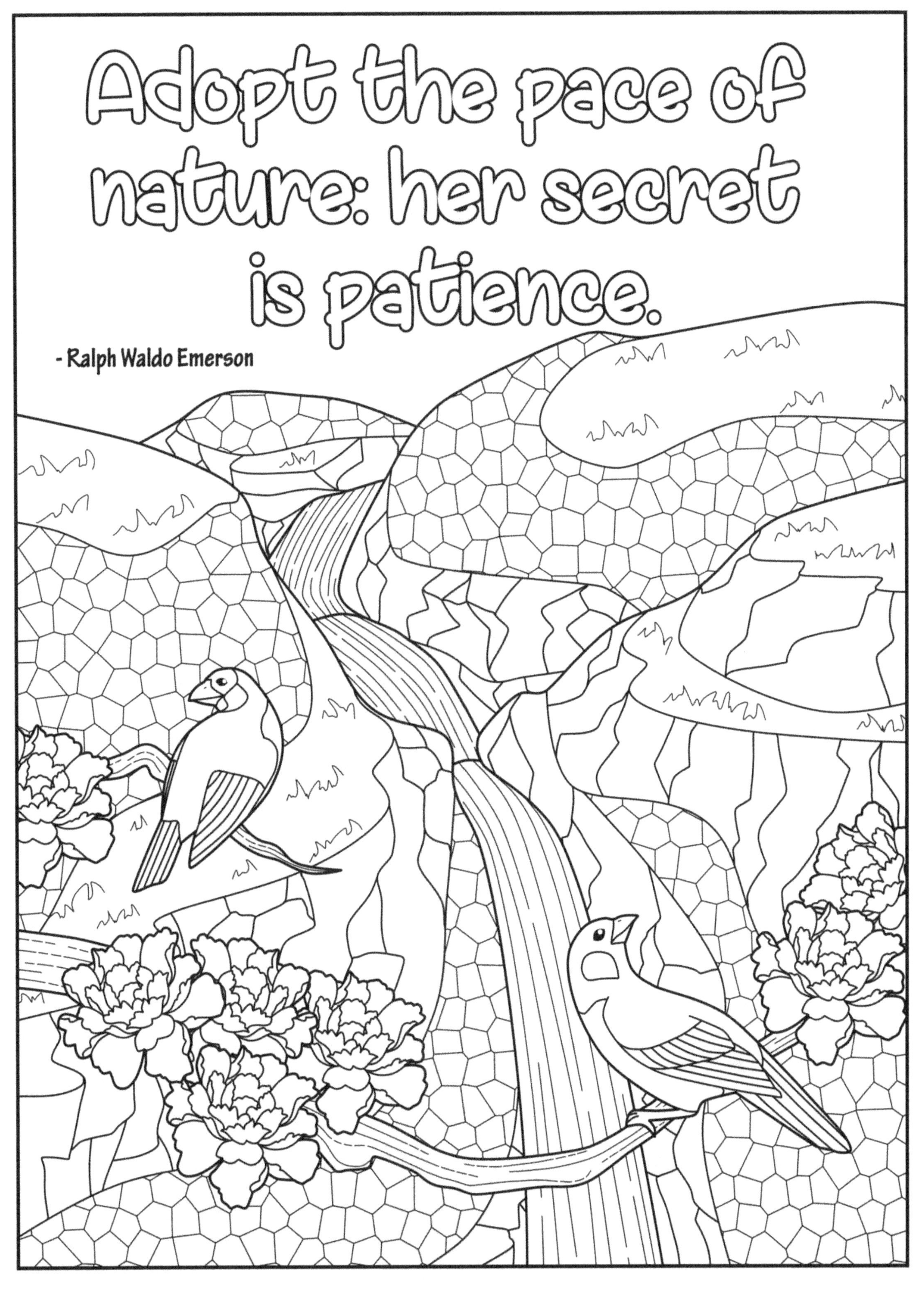

Adopt the pace of nature: her secret is patience.
- Ralph Waldo Emerson

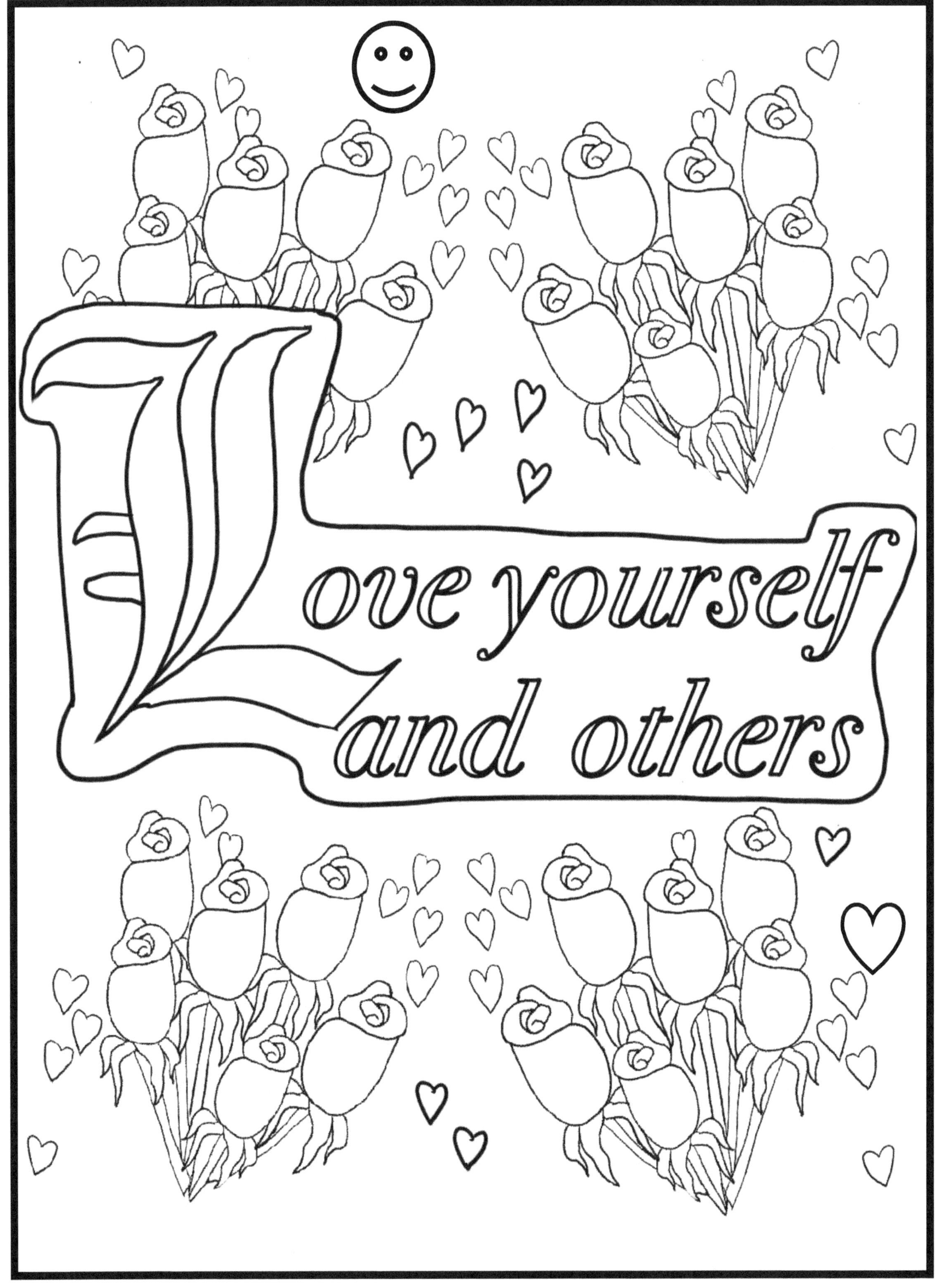

Love yourself
and others

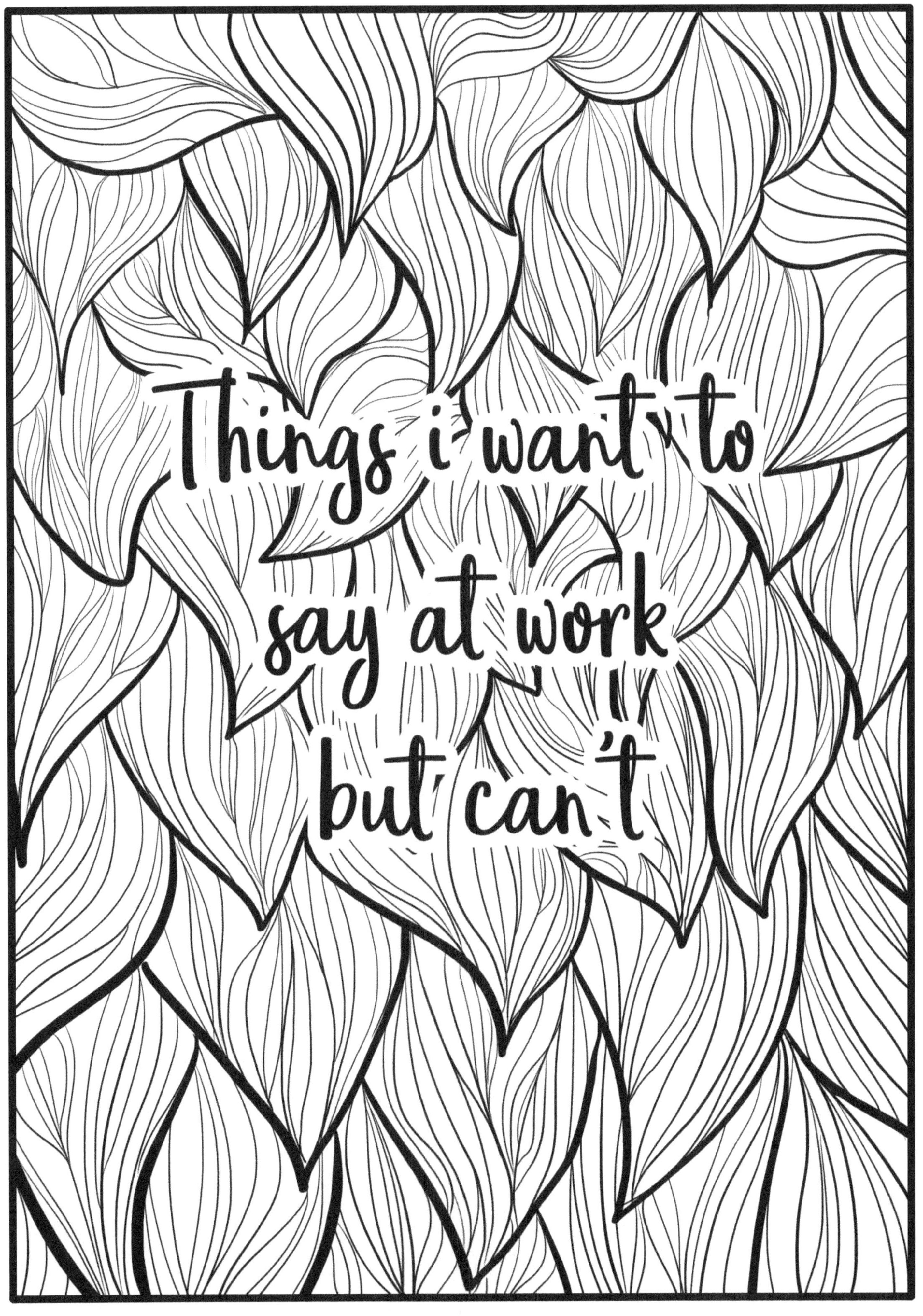
Things i want to
say at work
but can't

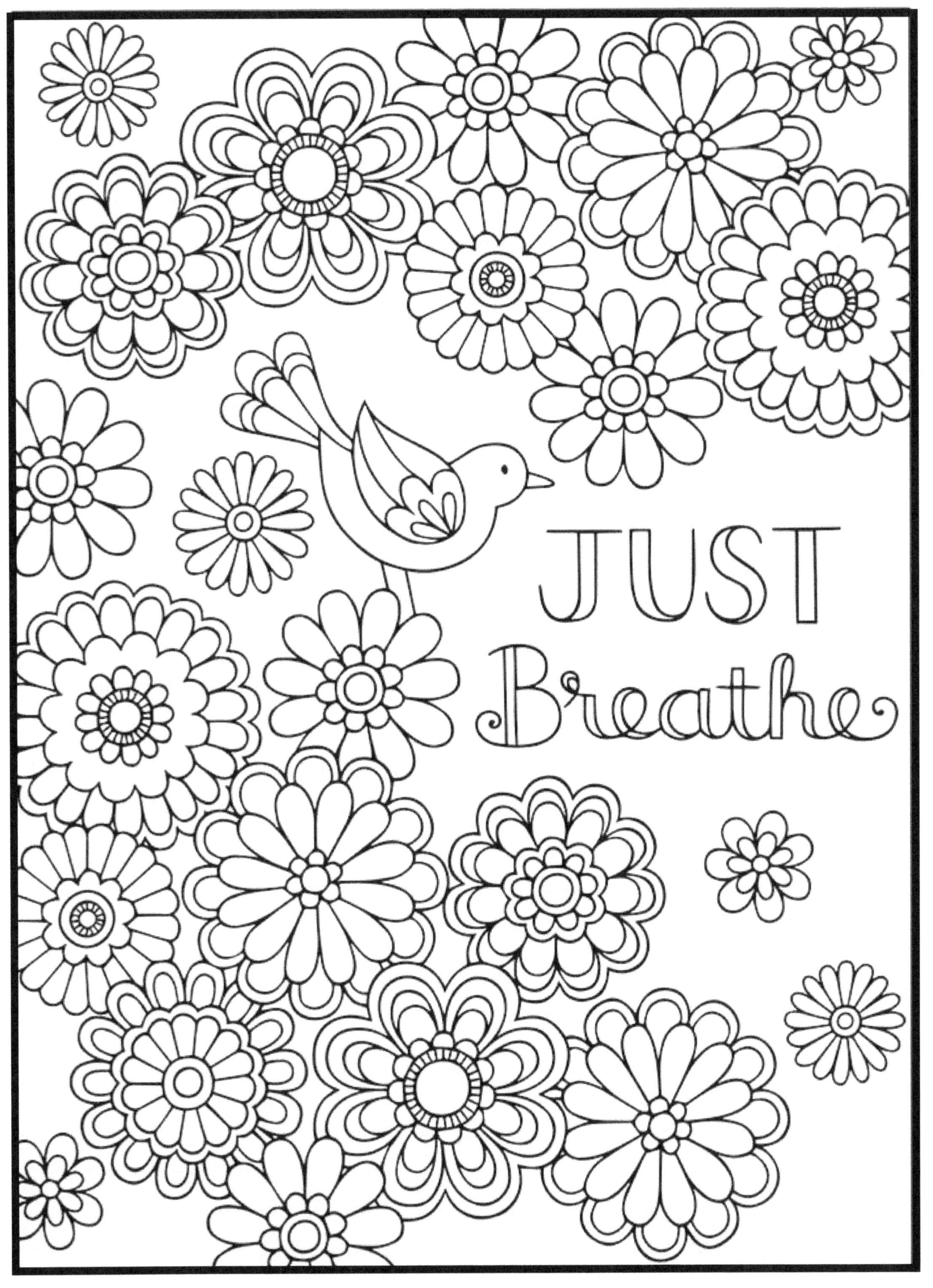
JUST
Breathe

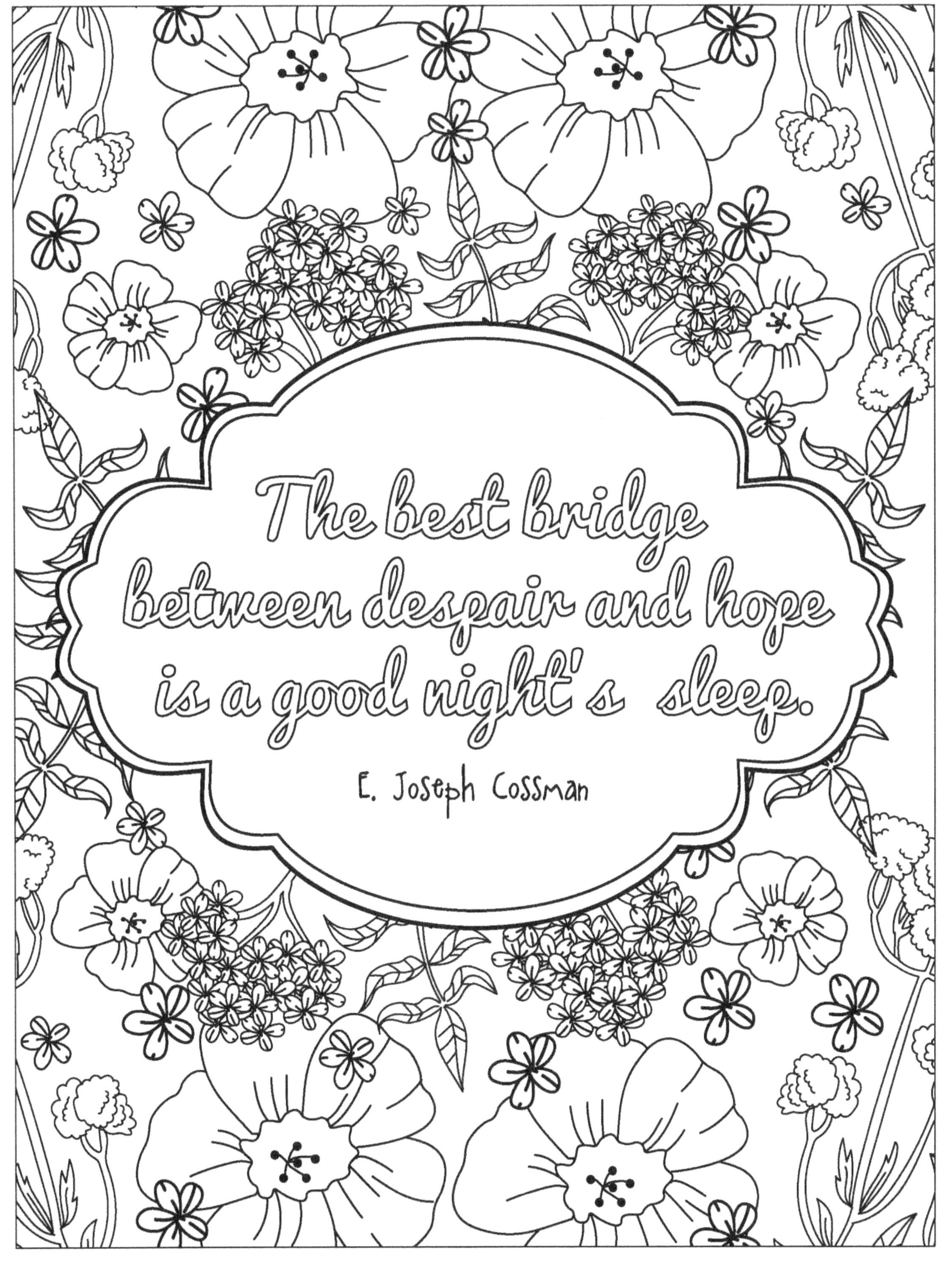

The best bridge
between despair and hope
is a good night's sleep.
E. Joseph Cossman

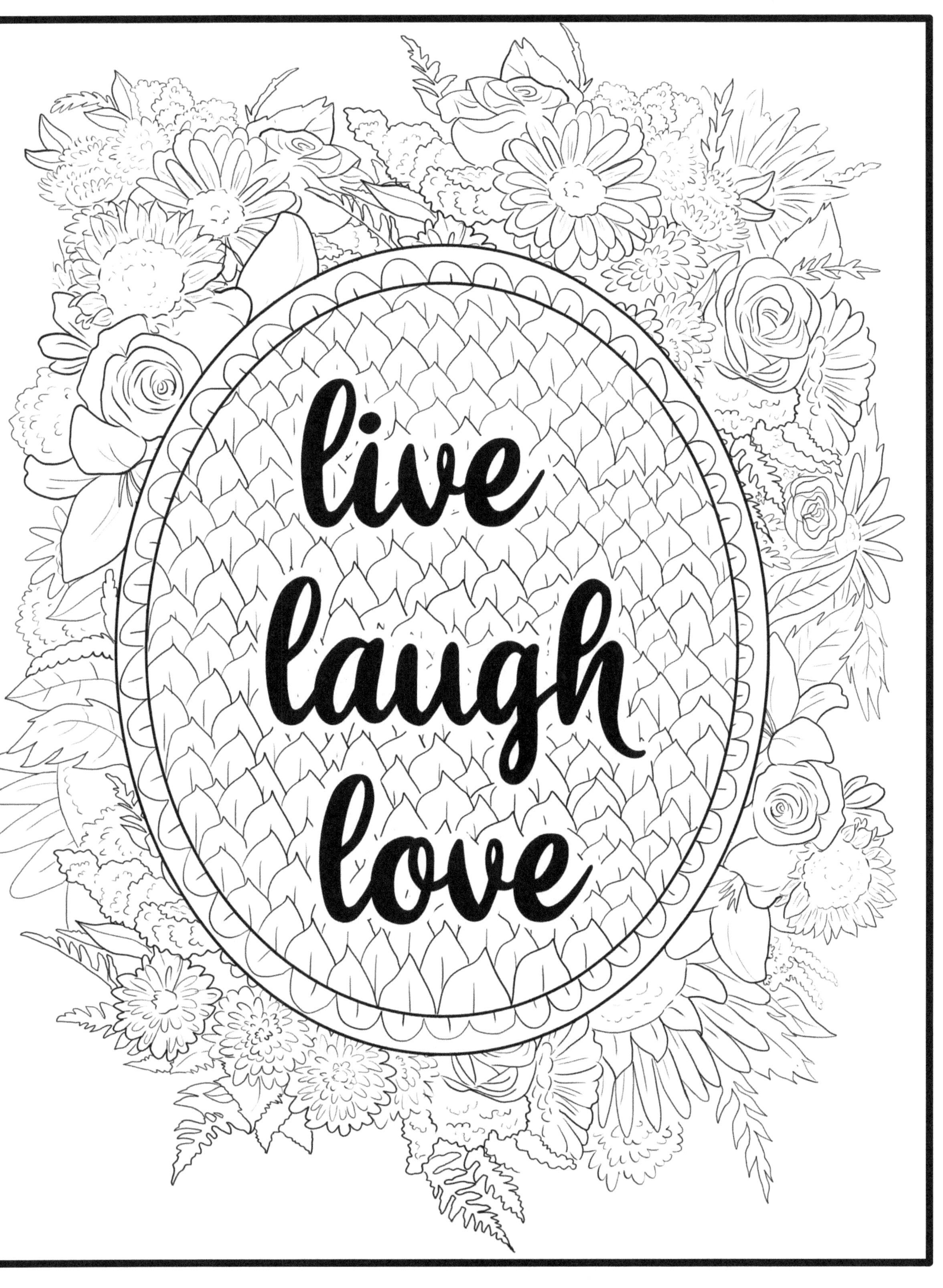

live
laugh
love

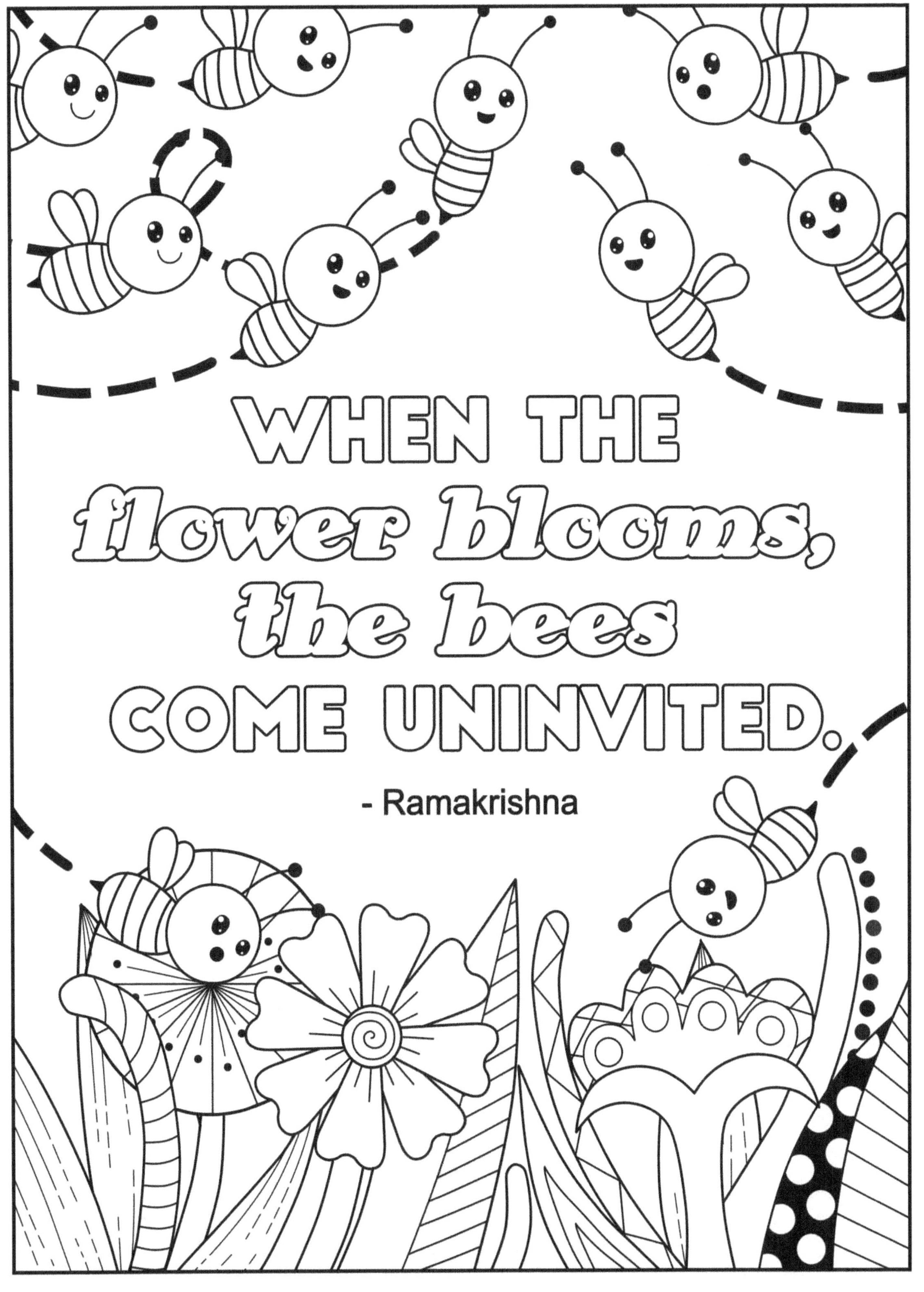

WHEN THE
flower blooms,
the bees
COME UNINVITED.
- Ramakrishna

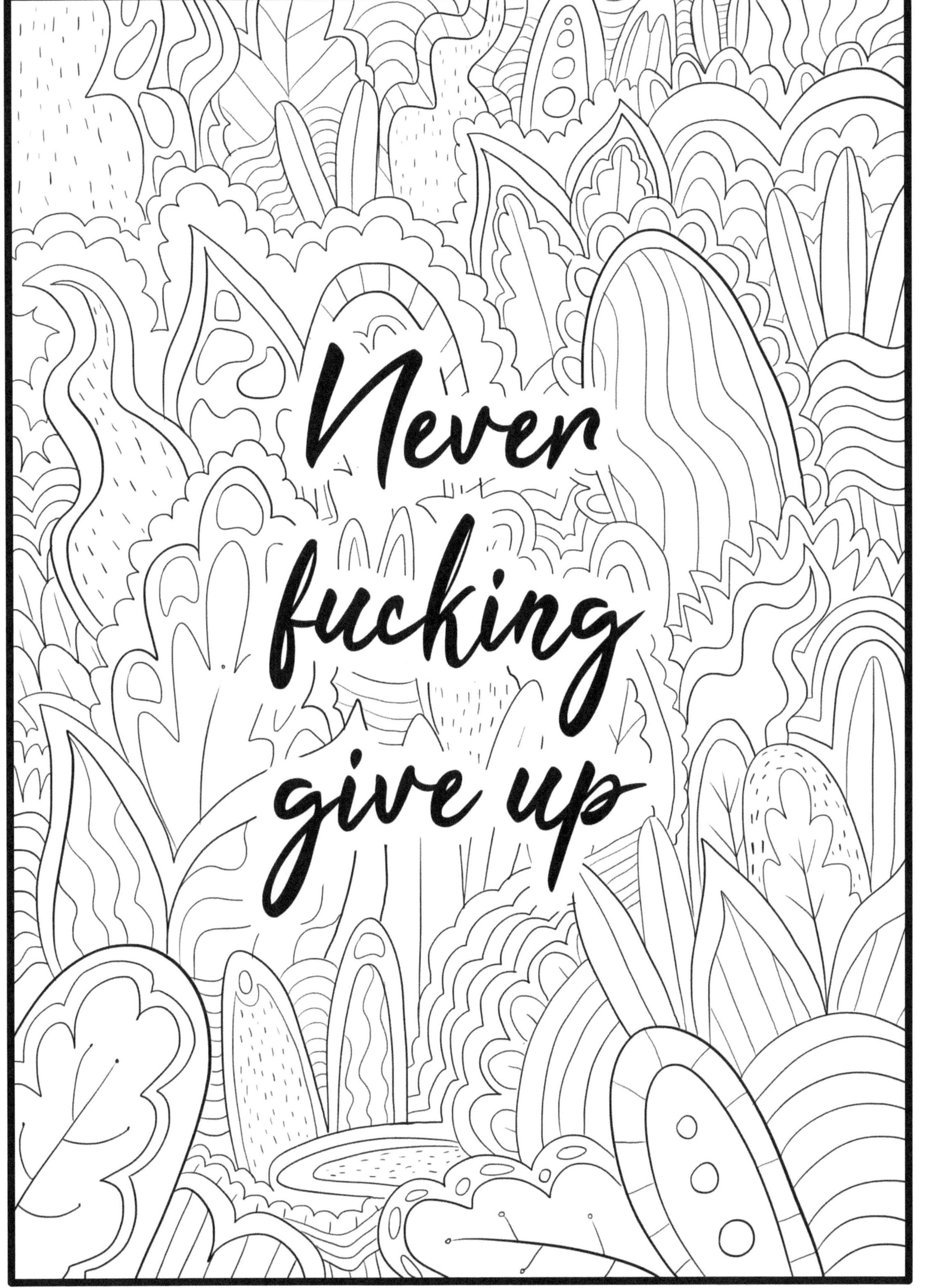
Never
fucking
give up

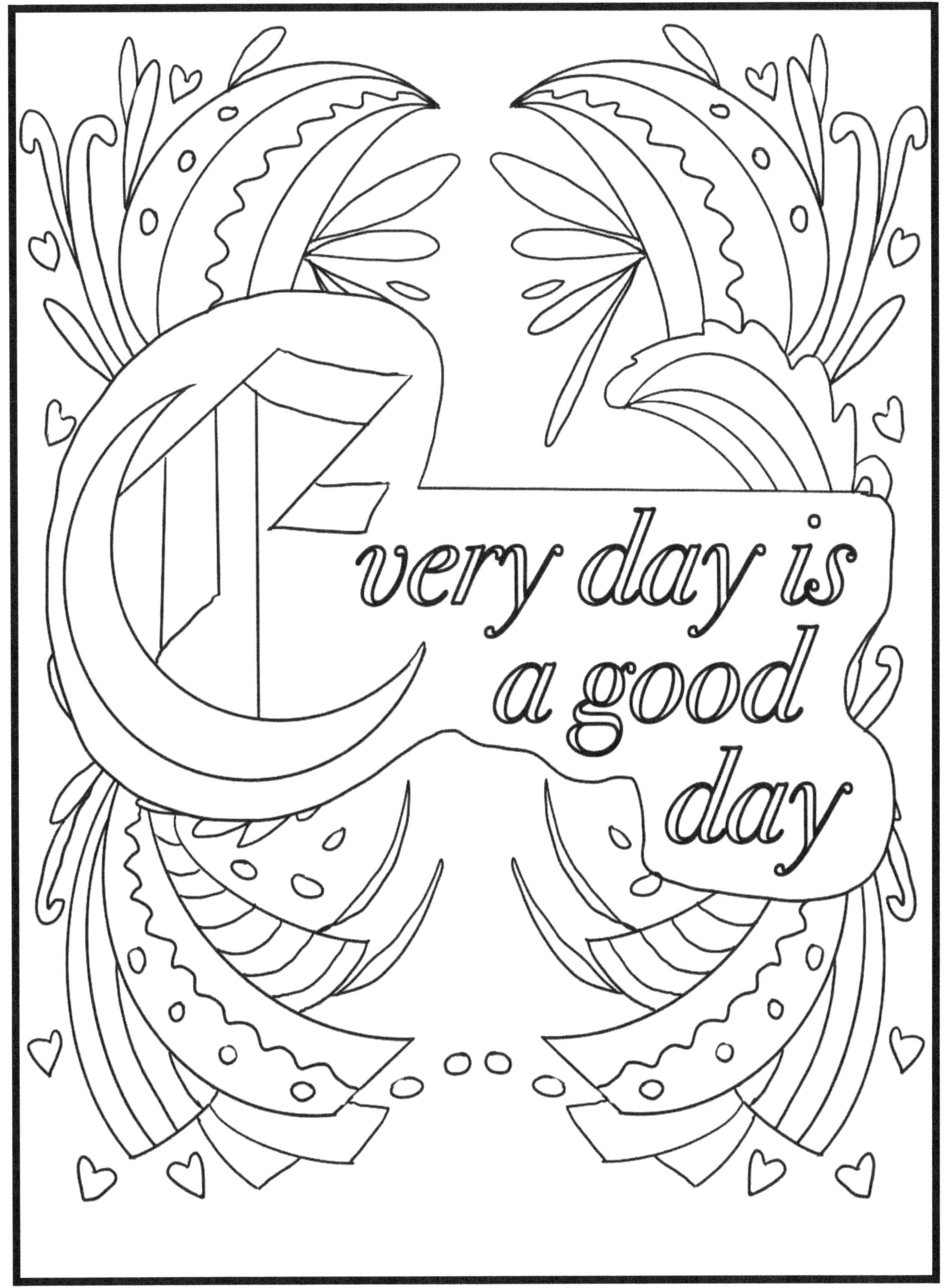

Every day is a good day

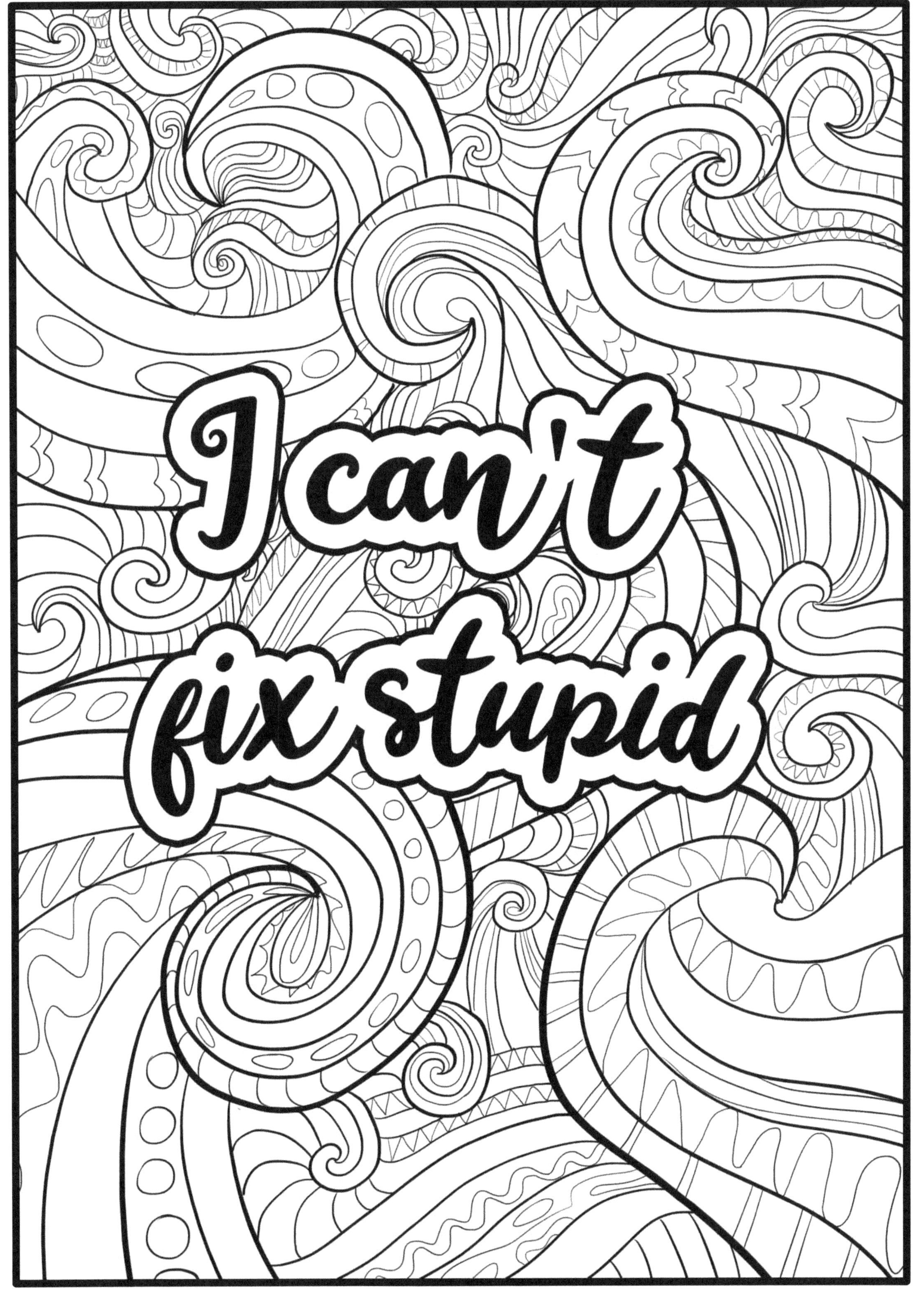

I can't
fix stupid

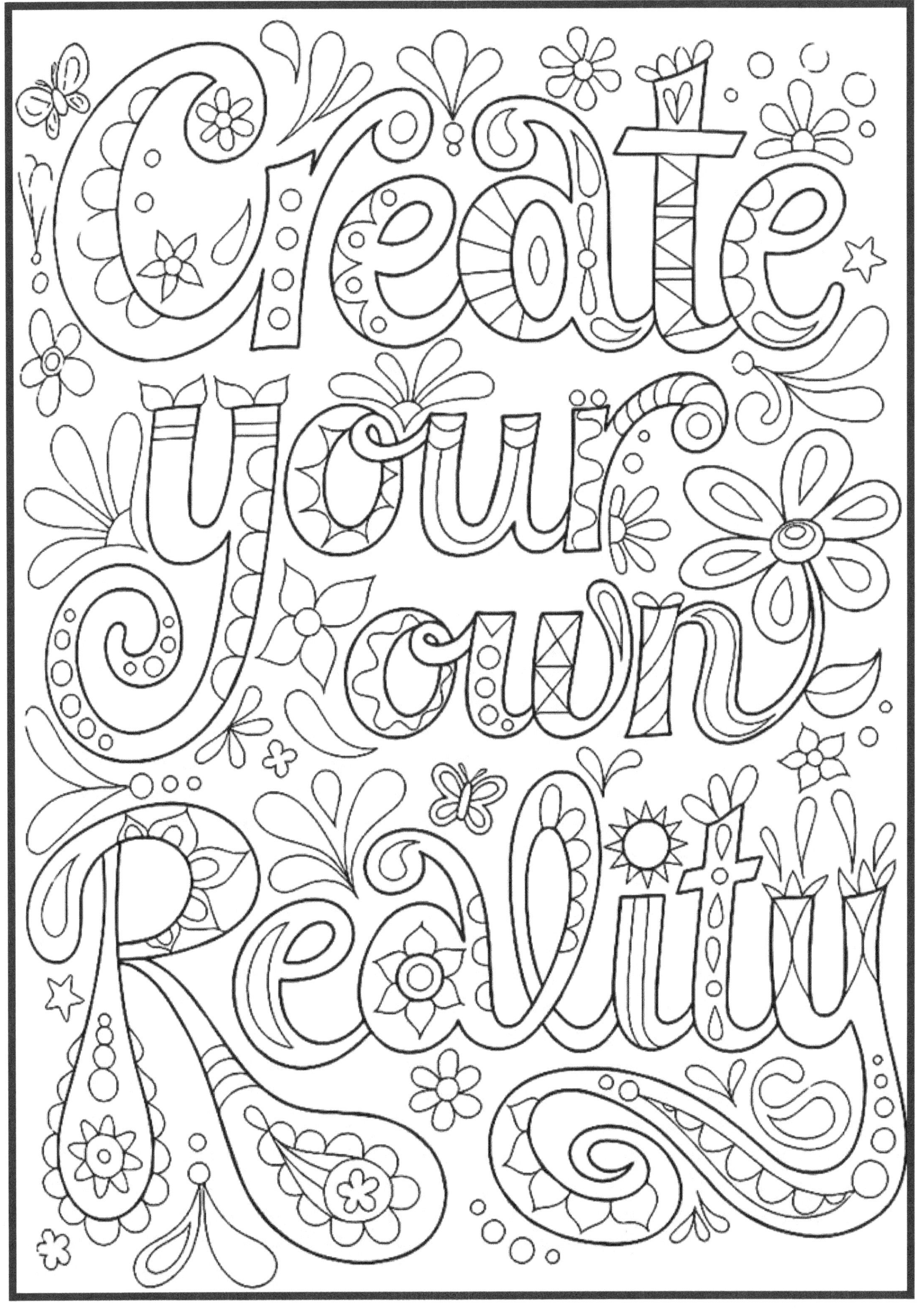

Create
your
own
Reality

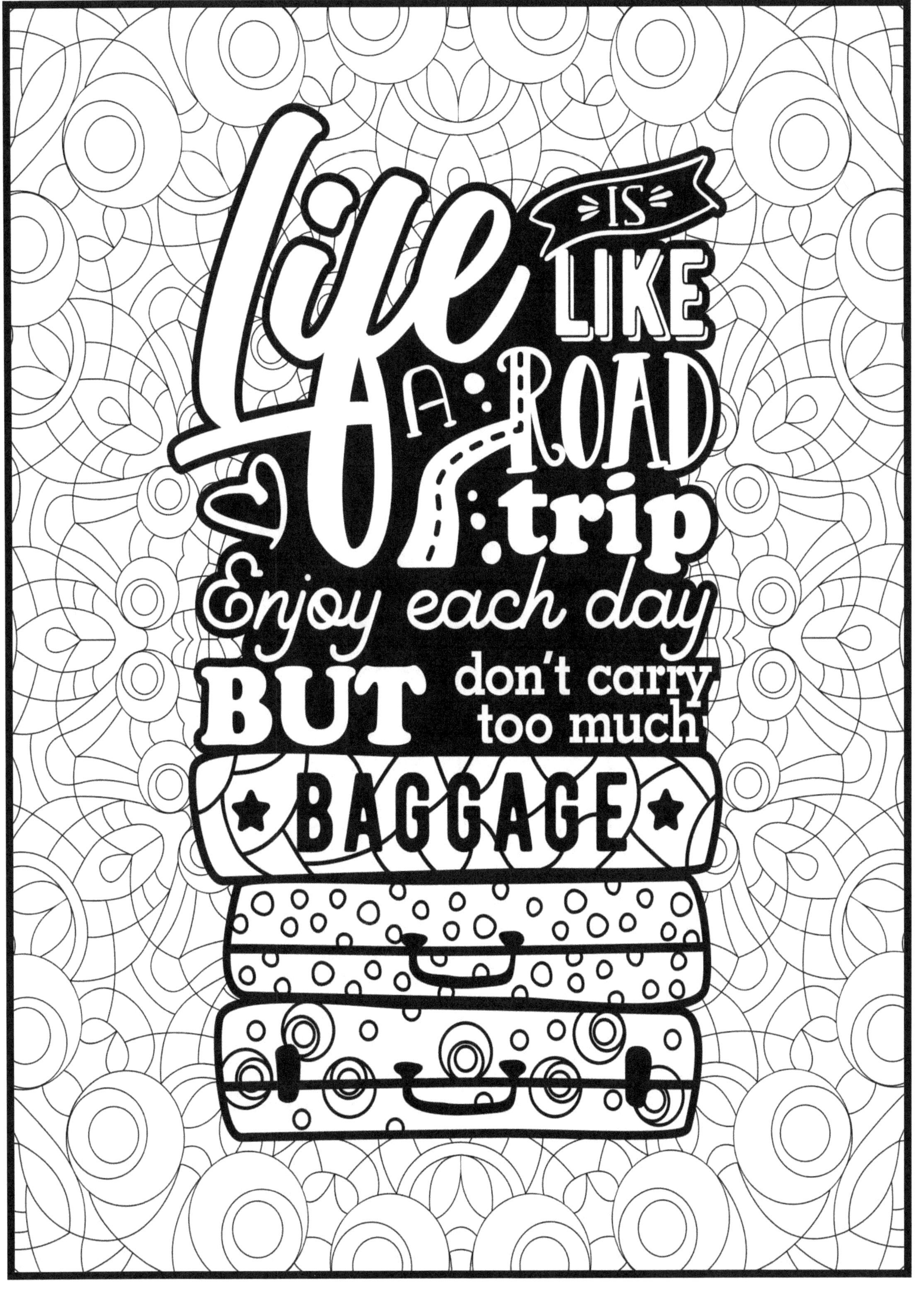

Life
IS
LIKE
A ROAD
trip
Enjoy each day
BUT don't carry too much
BAGGAGE

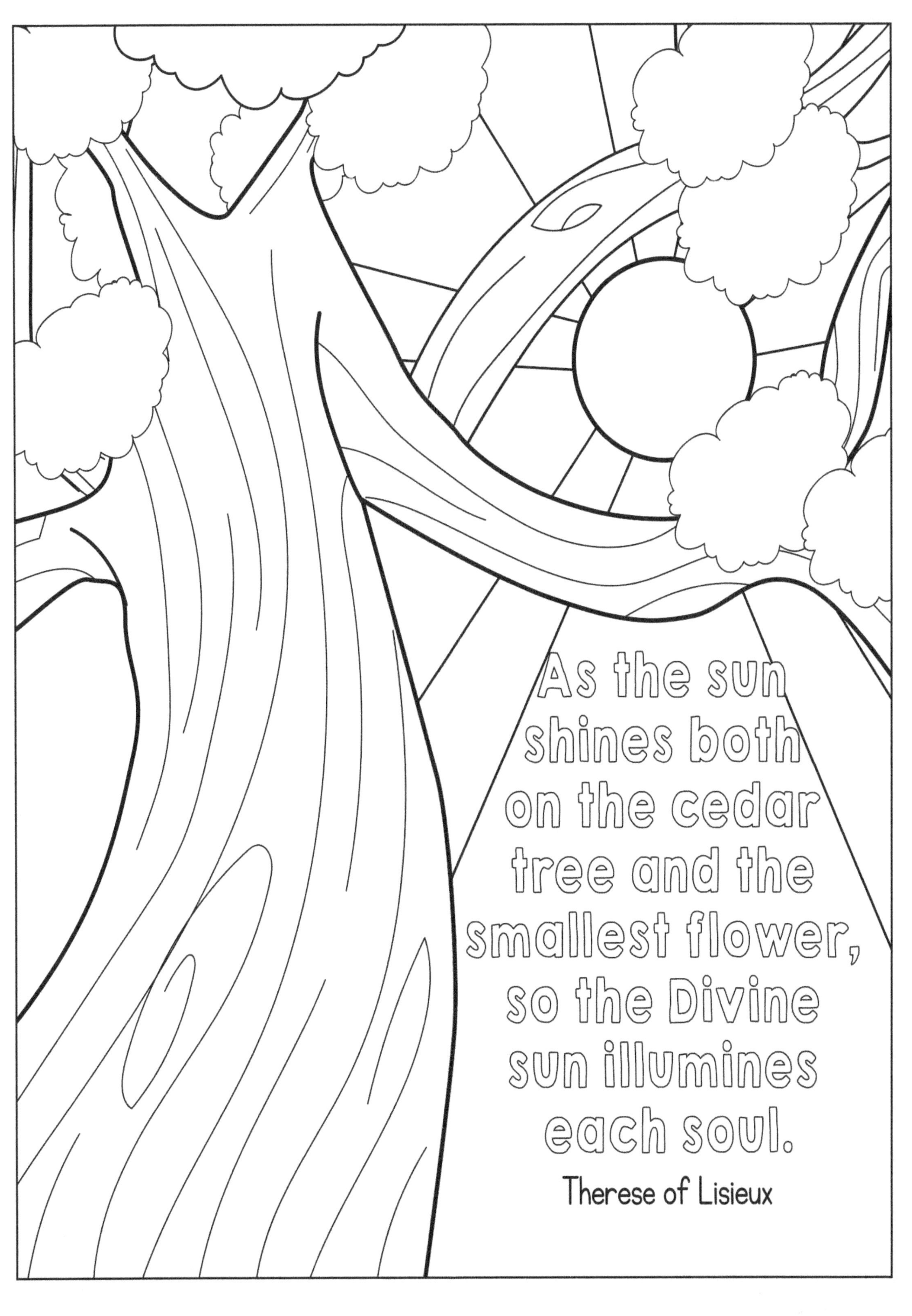

As the sun shines both on the cedar tree and the smallest flower, so the Divine sun illumines each soul.
Therese of Lisieux

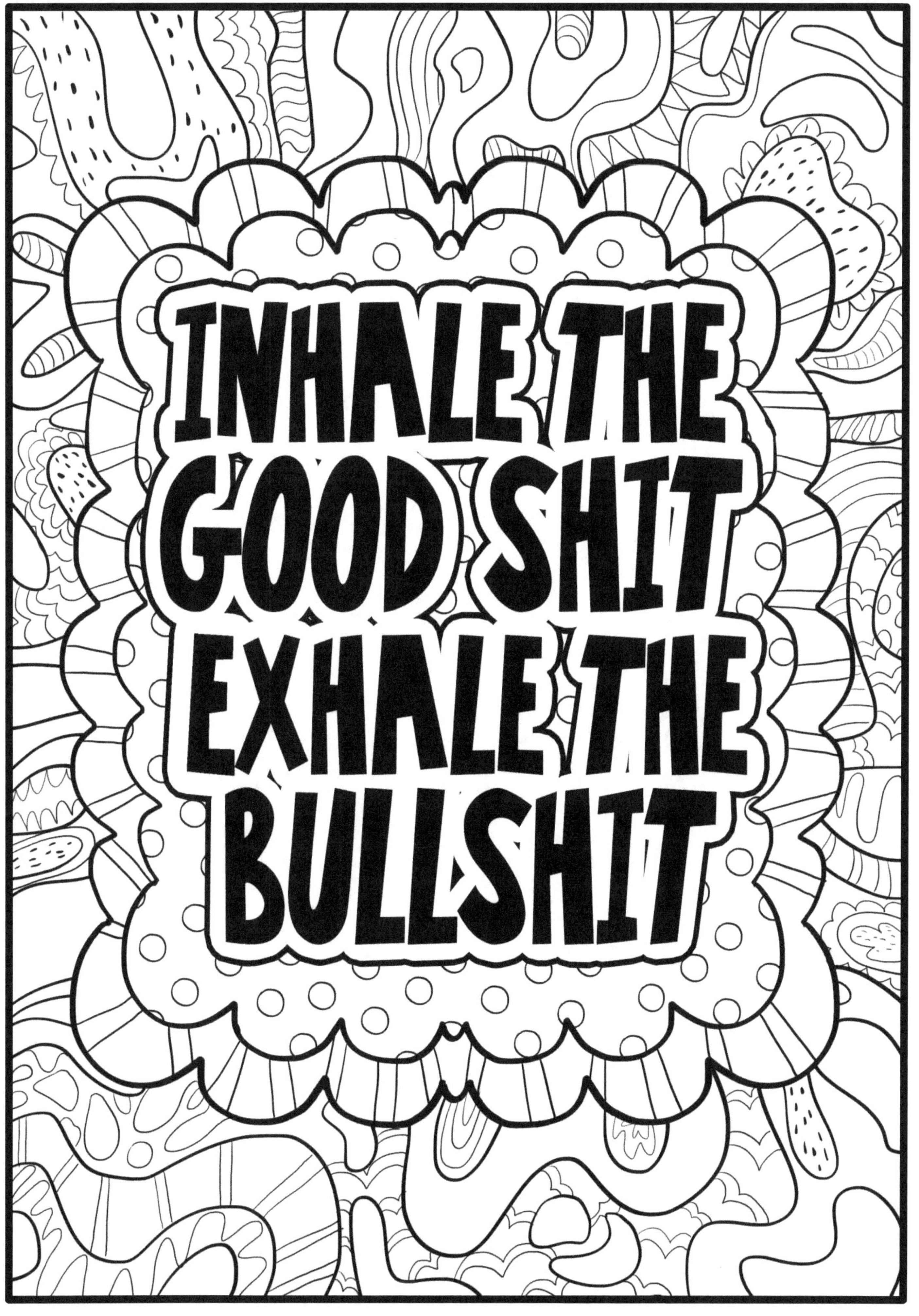

INHALE THE GOOD SHIT EXHALE THE BULLSHIT

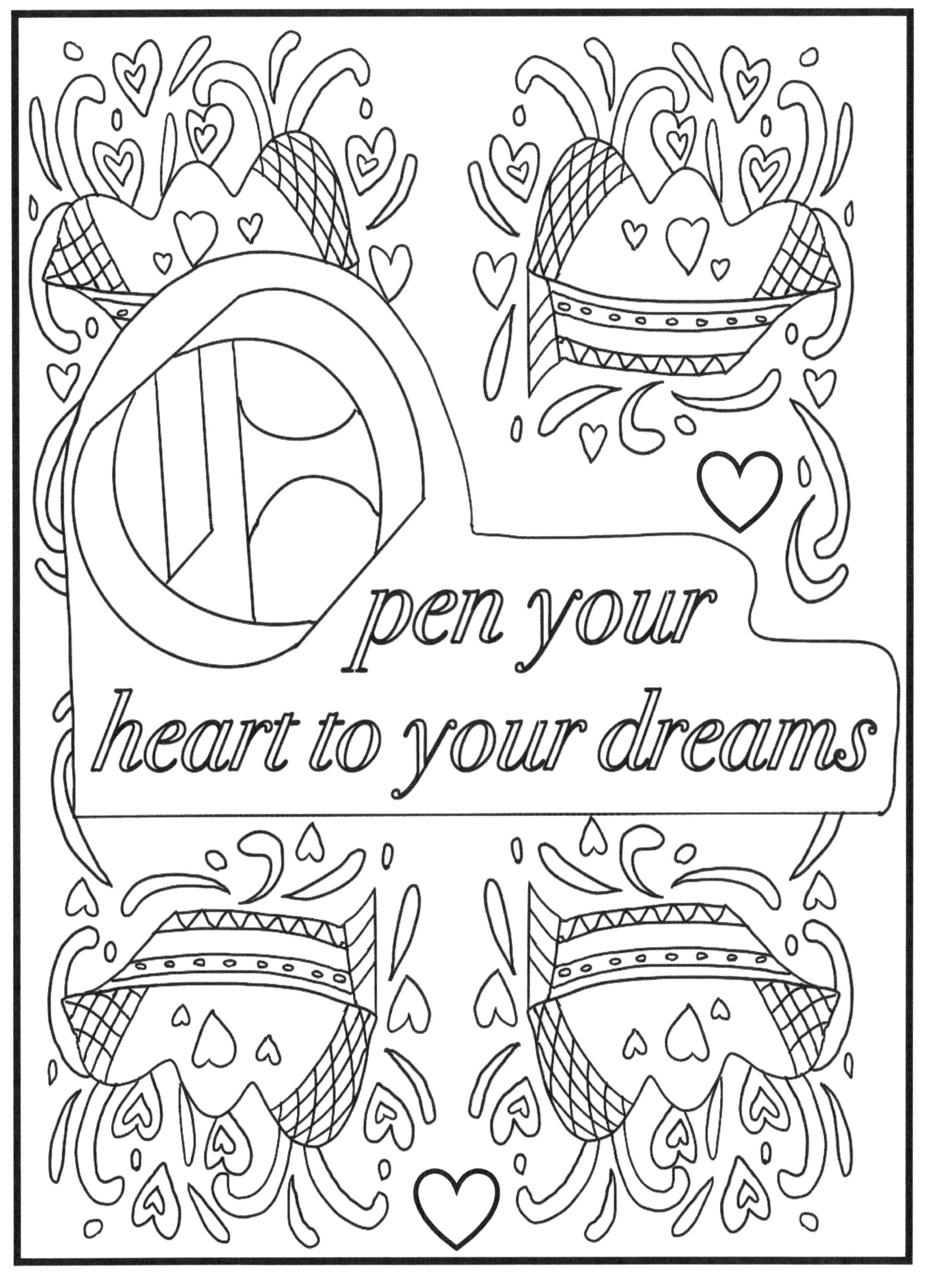

Open your
heart to your dreams

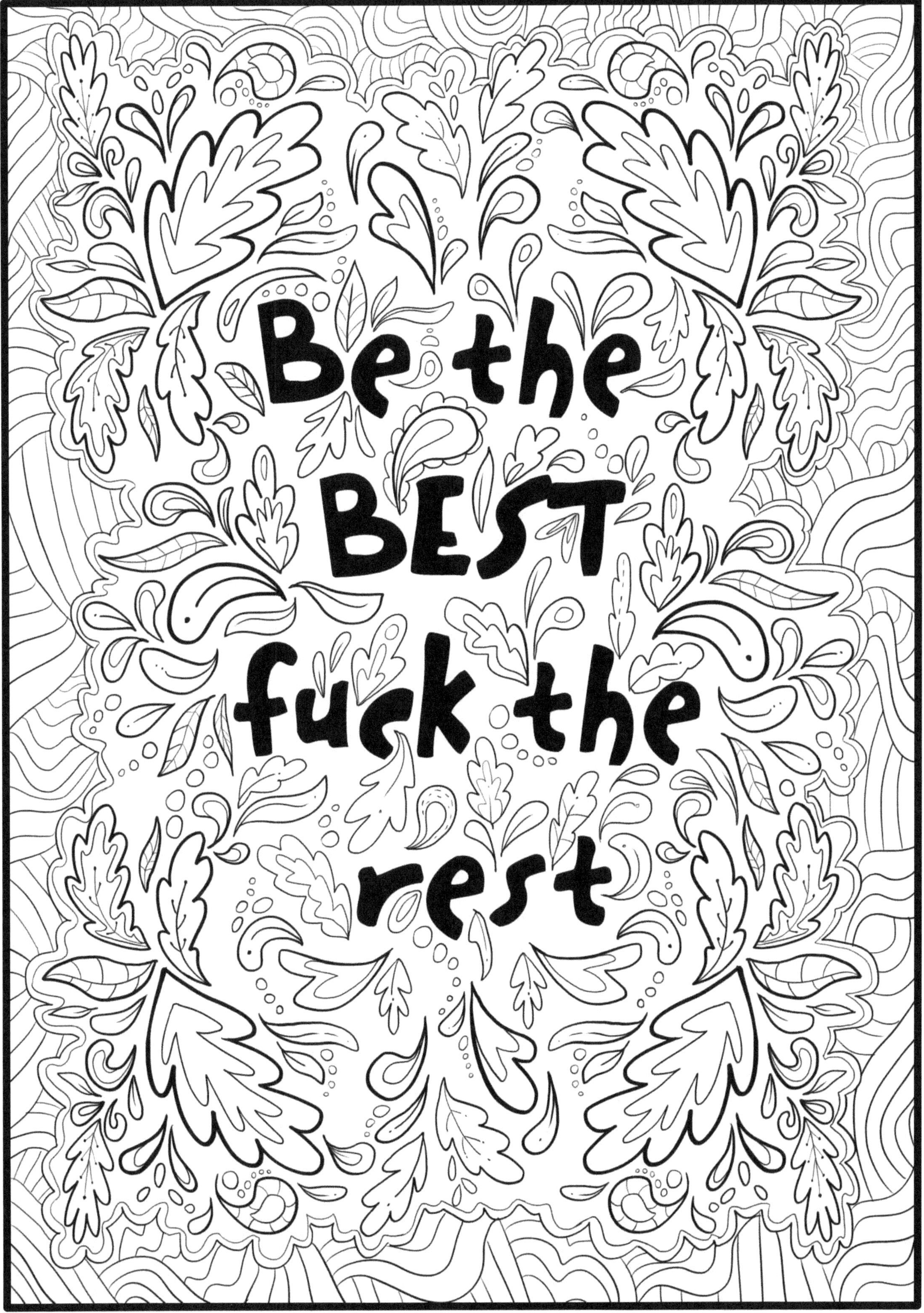

Be the
BEST
fuck the
rest

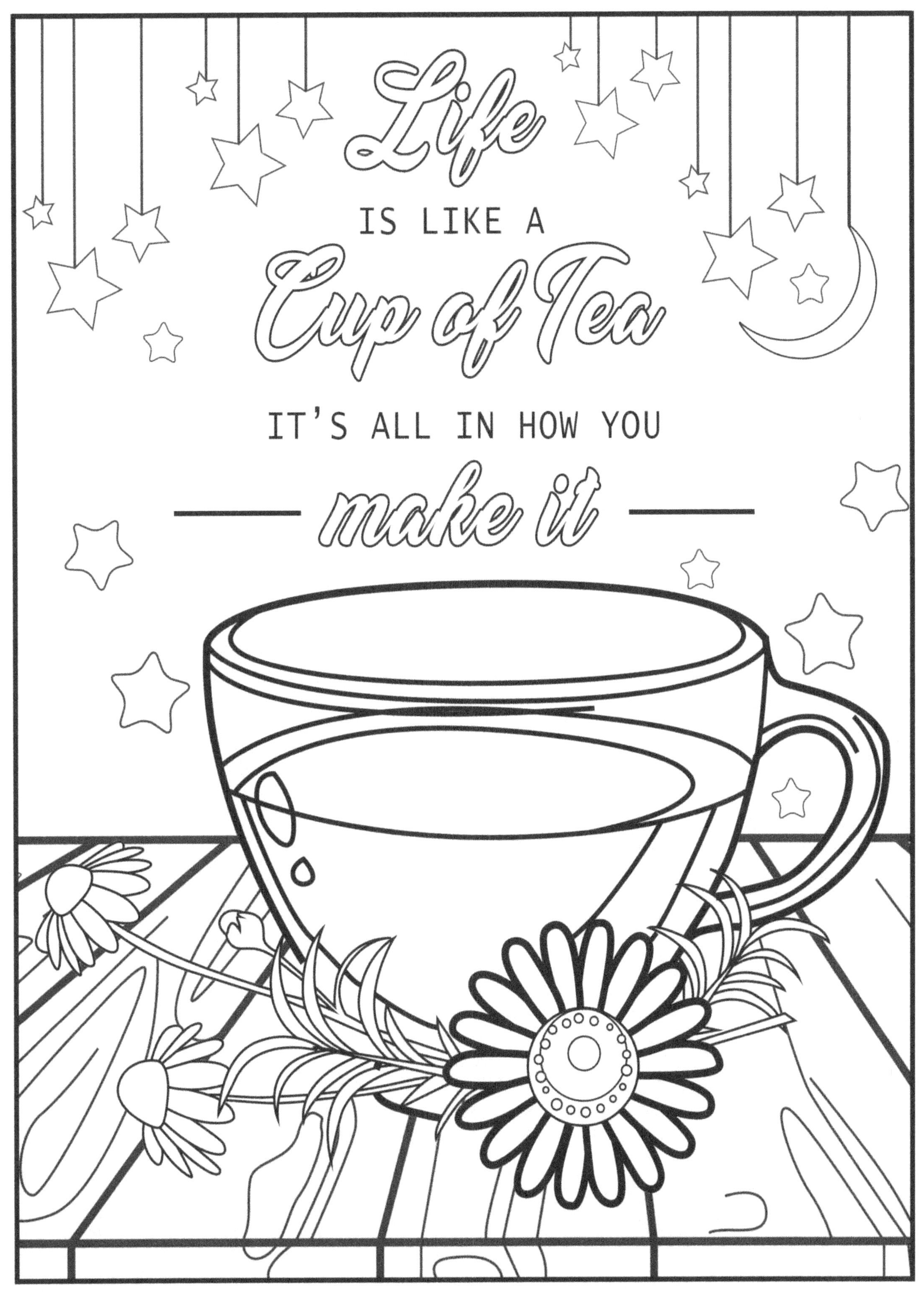

Life
IS LIKE A
Cup of Tea
IT'S ALL IN HOW YOU
make it

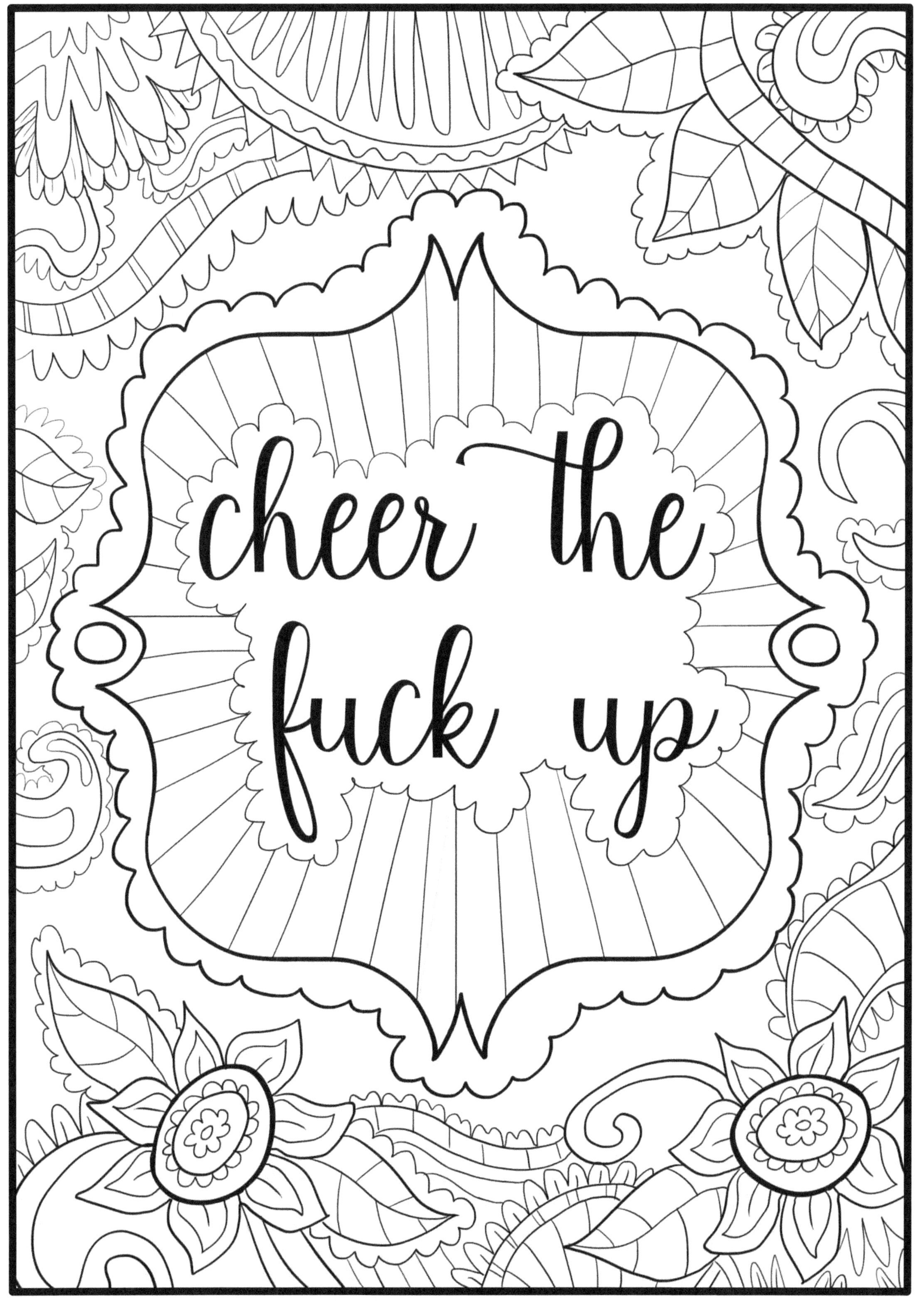

cheer the
fuck up

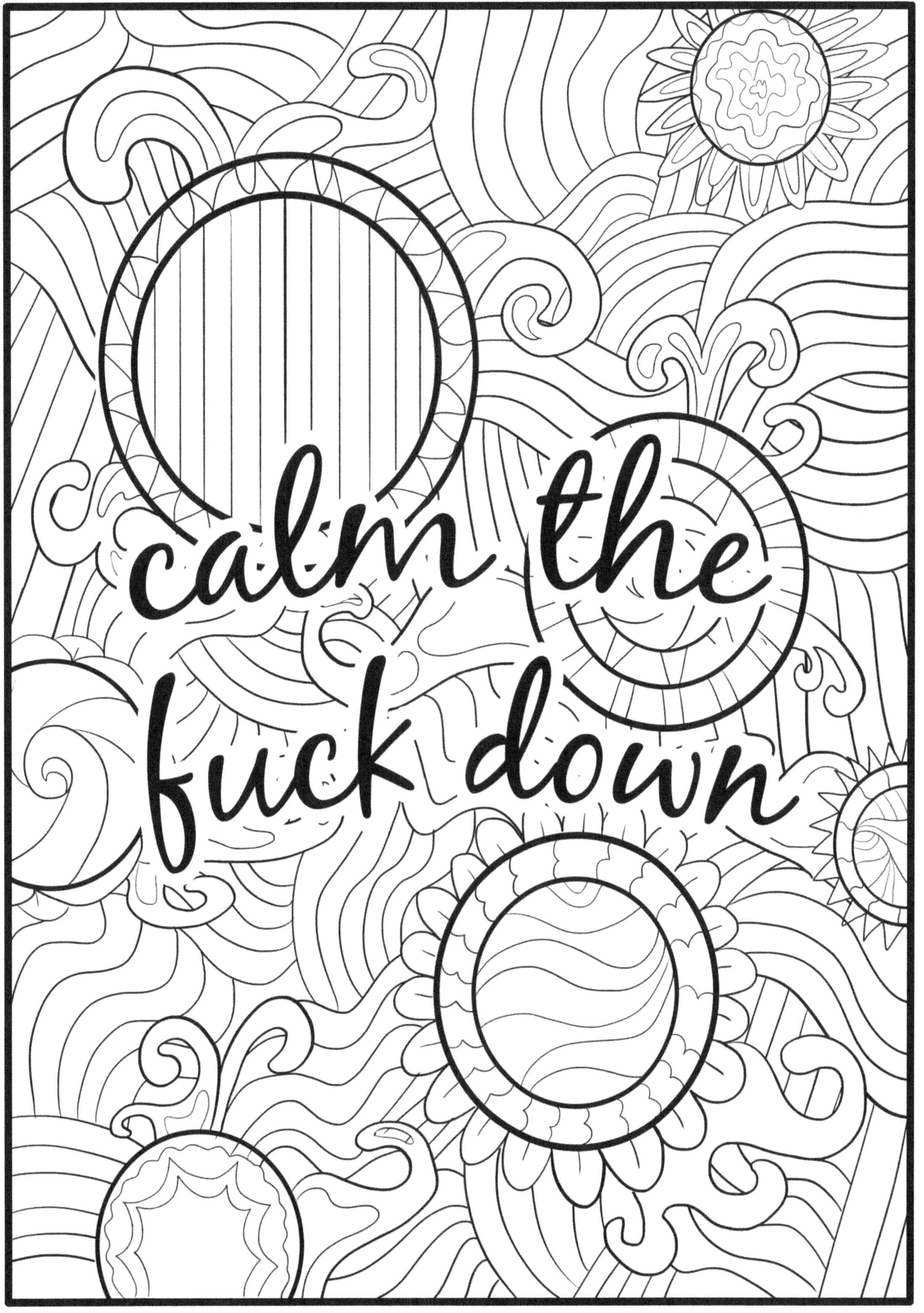

calm the
fuck down

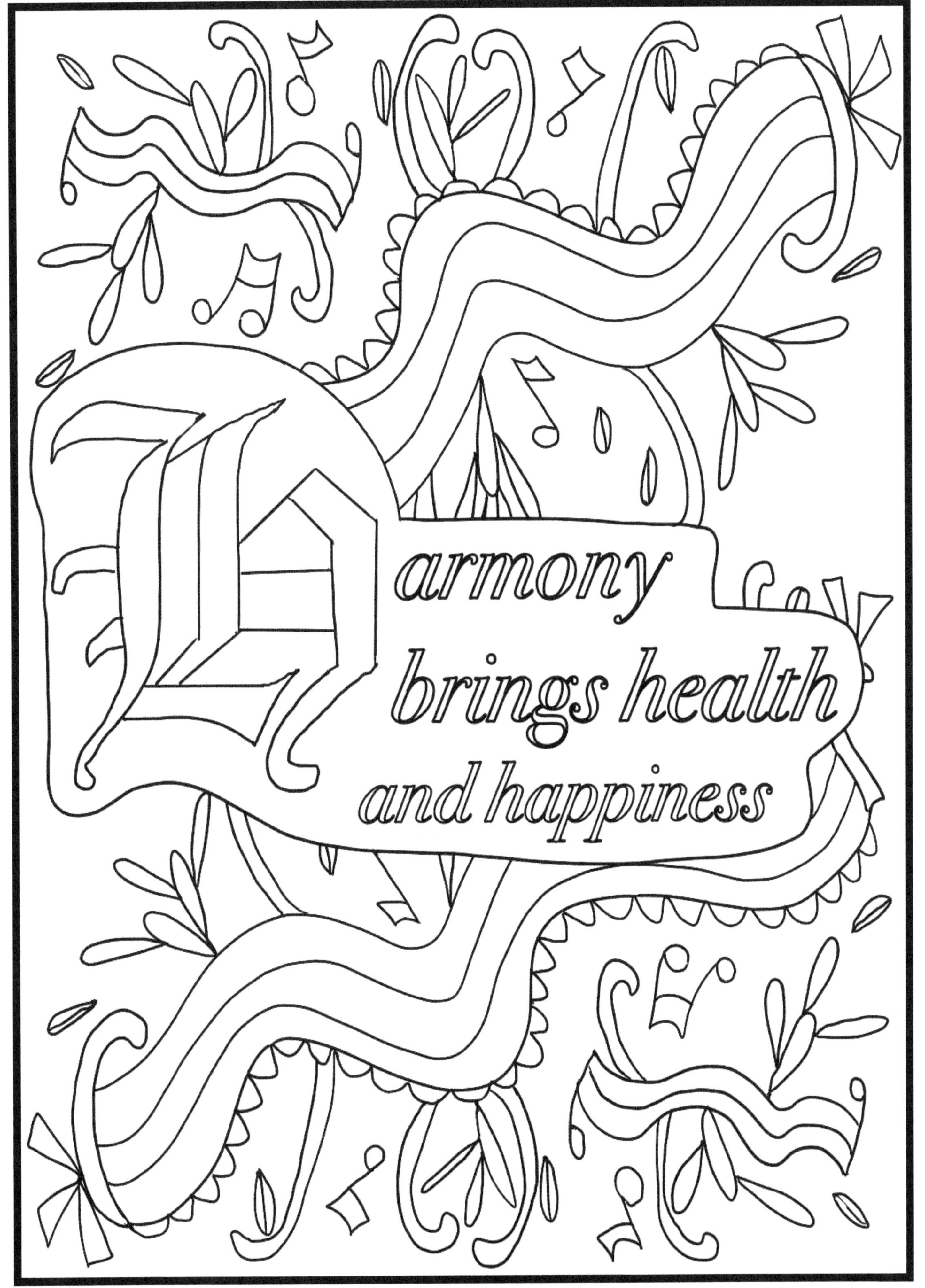

Harmony
brings health
and happiness

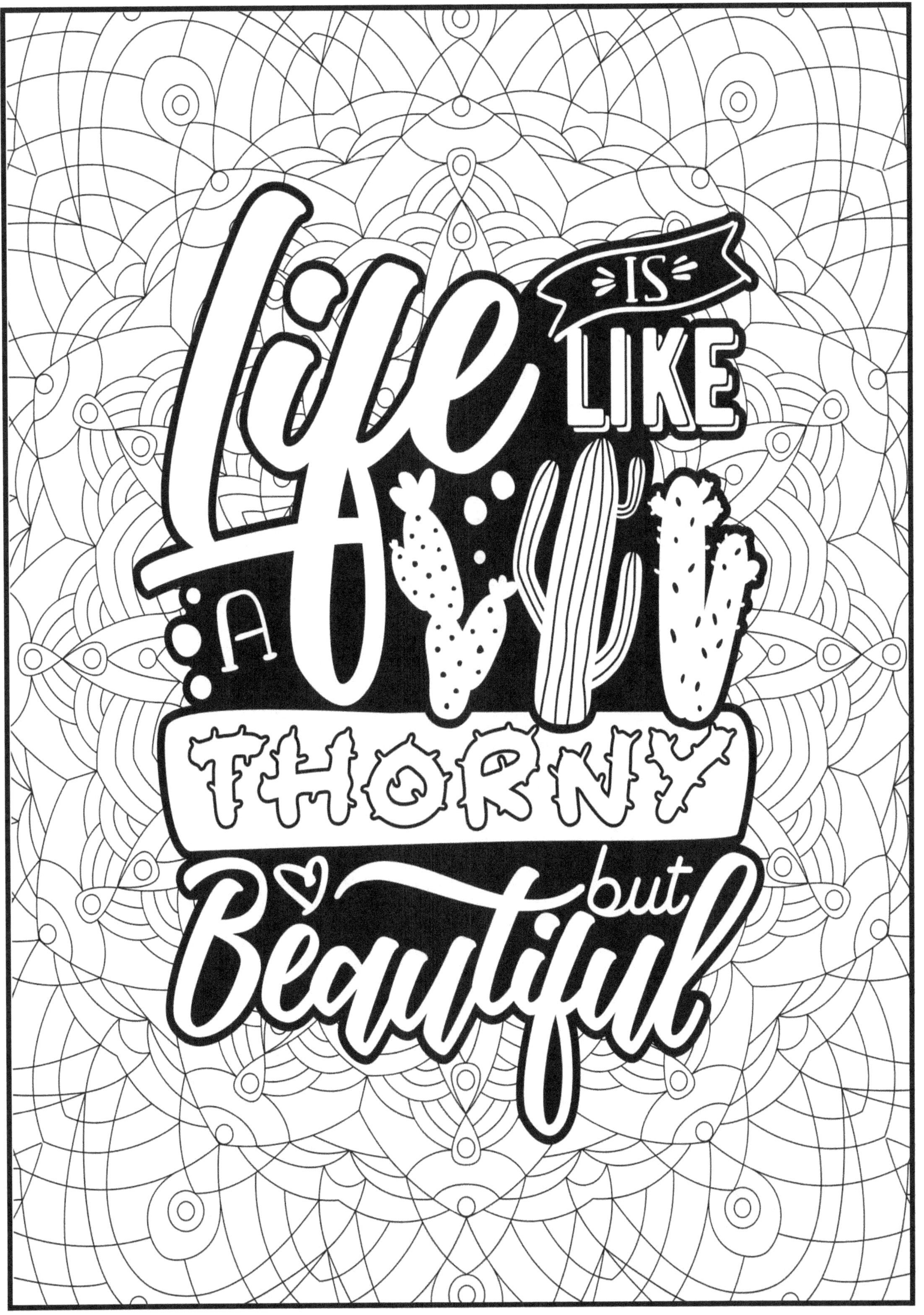

Life
IS
LIKE
A
THORNY
but
Beautiful